D0868252

Prayer, Laughter & Broccoli
Being There When Your Wife Has Breast Cancer

Peter J. Flierl, MSW

Alison Billings Flierl
Editor & Contributor

ISBN: 0-9745179-0-9

Witty Fools Productions
Los Angeles _ Greenwich
Copyright © 2004 Peter Flierl

Cover design courtesy of Byne Graphics

COMING FROM PETER FLIERL
The Ten Percent Solution

Dedication

This book is dedicated to Shirley Ann Billings
Flierl, my bride and my life partner, the mother
of my daughter, Alison, my lover, my business
partner and my best friend. Shirley was
diagnosed with an aggressive metastatic breast
cancer when she thought herself to be "too
young" and "too small" and at a time when we
had so much to live for. It was her courage,
faith, humor, persistence and joy that brought
Alison and me through this experience whole
and better for it.

Acknowledgements

I would like to thank my sister, Margaret Bennett, who is also a survivor, for her friendship and love since we were children together, and for her insights, support and encouragement during all of life's travails, and, in particular, during my writing of this book

I also wish to express my gratitude to Ray Melilllo, Ed Vicinanza, Joseph Locasio and Glenn Appleyard for teaching me to reach for the stars and to pursue my dreams. Lucy Hedrick, a true friend, showed me the way to writing as an avocation and Julia Cameron ignited my creative soul with *The Artist's Way* at a time when my soul definitely needed recharging.

Our family would like to acknowledge the love and support of many special friends and people who have helped us over the bumps and still do enrich our lives. This includes friends like Frank and Ellen Schigg, Bill and Jackie Hammock, the late Pat Brown, and Phyllis Finn. First Congregational Church and our friends and colleagues saw to it that we did not have to cook a meal from scratch for months after the start of Shirley's treatment, nor did we lack for child care. We are grateful.

Shirley and I are both grateful for the special love, comfort and support of Bart Crisafi and his first wife, the late Louisie Crisafi, who together set the standard for loving and living as a couple raising a family. Louise is up there looking after us.

Most of all, I'd like to thank my wife, Shirley Ann and my daughter, Alison for everything. They are my life.

Table of Contents

Our Odyssey

Our family's incredible healthcare odyssey began the summer of 1982 in Winter Harbor, Maine, when Shirley Ann took part in a hokey Lobster Festival parade. She felt something in her breast, attributed it to a pulled muscle from aerobics in the parade, or perhaps the lumpy horse hair mattresses we slept on and made love on. Her woman's intuition knew better, but denial is powerful.

The inexorable movement toward diagnosis and treatment began in the Fall, starting with her internist, Jeffrey Weinberger, then a local gynecologist followed by a man who was about to become her surgeon, Phil McWhorter, a good surgeon and a friend. The final step was seeing her oncologist, Dickerman Hollister, Jr., a Renaissance man who, along with the late Joseph Murphy, her radiologist and radiation therapist, saved her life.

The initial diagnosis was devastating. "We're too young. I don't want her to die. I can't live without her." The Kubla Ross stages setting in: denial, anger, acceptance. I do not want to be a single Dad raising a child on my own. God did not mean for it to be that way. And yet that's what we were facing or I was feeling.

Shirley knew from her conversations with Phil and Dick that she had the worst of the worst possible scenarios. Extensive lymph node involvement, an aggressive metastatic form of breast cancer with a very poor prognosis. Phil punched me in the stomach with his words following her surgery: "The tumor was too large and too deep into the chest wall for me to completely remove it."

Shirley would need extensive chemotherapy, hormone therapy and radiation treatment. The world was turning dark. A year or so following her surgery, Shirley commiserated with former First Lady Betty Ford on the dance floor at a charity ball in New York. That was when I first learned of or was able to take in that many lymph nodes were involved. I never shared Phil's words with her until year's later.

Our first sit down together with Dick Hollister was a moment to remember. We were "playing for all the marbles." Did we want to save Shirley or leave open the option of additional children in the future? Our joint response took a nanosecond. Dick walked us through his proposed regimen or course of treatment: six months of chemotherapy and hormone therapy, followed by six weeks of radiation, and then another six months of the same strong chemotherapy and hormone therapy. He also offered us sources for second opinions in New

York or Boston, followed by telling us he would take our case and his proposed treatment protocol to Yale-New Haven Hospital for review. A no-brainer for both of us then and in retrospect.

Medicine is built on relationship and trust. A good physician is still a hands-on healer, despite all the technology and resources to be brought to bear. We opted for Dick. We opted for and received life. Precious, precious life and health.

Tell her you love her.

In a marriage or any intimate relationship, silence is not golden. The strong silent type need not apply for the position of husband, lover, best friend, confidante, caregiver and supporter of a woman with breast cancer. Your bride, your wife, needs and wants to hear from you. Actions may speak louder than words, and you may take all the right actions, but speaking words brings comfort, reassurance and knowledge of your inner feelings. She cannot read your mind. Being there for her is more than physical or economic security. Words have meaning. And the three most important words in the English language at this time, at this moment, when you together face her mortality, are: "I love you."

The late Louise Crisafi, a saint here on Earth always giving of herself for others in need, taught me this lesson on the Friday Shirley had her biopsy and was diagnosed, having opted for the then new two-step process. This meant we knew on Friday that she would have a mastectomy on Monday, a weekend together, scared, anxious, and frightened. For Shirley, confronting death and loss of a part of her womanhood. For me, at a loss, not knowing what to do or what to say.
Louise was an American Cancer Society Reach to Recovery volunteer devoted to helping other

women facing breast cancer diagnosis and treatment. She was a good friend. When I asked Louise what to do feeling as helpless and overwhelmed as I was, she said simply: "Tell her you love her." I was off to the races. I spent the weekend saying those magic, powerful words over and over, as frequently as possible, perhaps more than I had done in weeks, months or years previously.

A year or so later in a television talk show featuring three women with breast cancer, including Louise, Shirley reminisced about how verbal I had become that fateful weekend. Those words brought comfort and made a difference. Say, "I love you." It works. And I hope I am doing so as much today.

Be faithful. Be monogamous.

We do not hear espoused or celebrated often enough the value and benefits of faithfulness, fidelity and monogamy. Nor do we hear of the sacred nature of marriage and its profound role in the social contract. A long term, monogamous relationship is exquisitely intimate.

A good friend, a woman, said of my views on monogamy: "How quaint." As in charming, old fashioned, unusual or unfamiliar, even strange. And then I look at our role models, Shirley's parents, Art and Marge, married for more than 62 years. That is the goal. We find in it our deepest nature, our essential and fundamental selves. We become acutely perceptive of each other in a relationship that is intense and keen. It is as delicate and beautiful as a snowflake, as hard and lustrous as a diamond.

As a man, you will understand with certainty that your wife truly completes you in every way: physically, emotionally, and spiritually. You owe it to her and yourself to develop the depth of understanding brought on only by being faithful for life. God meant us as marriage partners to be one together for life. Swans do it, so can we.

Say "Yes"

We all know the joke about Moses and the tribes of Israel wandering for 40 years in the desert after their miraculous escape from bondage in Egypt. It took 40 long years to reach the land of milk and honey, the Promised Land. And why, why did it take so long? Moses was a man. He refused to ask for directions. Ten Commandments, maybe; asking for help, never.

If you're married or even dating a man for any length of time, you've spent time in a car lost. You suggest, perhaps timidly and quietly, that it might be a good idea to stop and ask for directions. He is offended. He, after all, is a man. He has a good, no, a great sense of direction. That will become apparent to you, a mere woman with no sense of direction, momentarily. The moments tick by. He is becoming exasperated. Finally, in disgust, he pulls into a gas station and asks for help. It pains him to do so.

Louise Crisafi taught me to accept help when I asked her what to do knowing that Shirley and I were facing her cancer together, a cancer we had little hope of beating. Her advice was powerful and insightful. When someone, anyone, asks if they can do anything to help, say: "Yes." Friends, neighbors, colleagues and others want to be there for you and for themselves. I know, I know. You're a man and never ask for help, not even simple directions. Understand that the people asking to help need your "Yes" as much as you. It gives them some sense of being able to do something positive about this insidious disease that seems beyond their control.

Shirley and I were blessed. We did not have to cook a meal for 3-4 months following her surgery thanks to the chicken dishes, casseroles, lasagnas and other assorted goodies constantly flowing to our front door. Need a brief childcare stint for our daughter, Alison, it would be there. Thank you in particular First Congregational Church in Old Greenwich. Thank you special friends, particularly Betsy, who taught me I could get through anything, even this. You are a healing church. You were and are true friends. Your love, prayers and support made a difference for all three of us in our recovery.

Ask for help. Say "yes" when it's offered. You'll be better for it and so will those seeking to help.

Humor Heals

Norman Cousins taught the country this lesson many years ago and we are often reminded of this truth. We know that the act of laughing is healing. It makes us feel better and helps us get better. It is very easy to take ourselves in particular and our careers much too seriously.

Our close friends have experienced our occasional over-the-top, out of control laughing, true guffaws. Can anything feel better? You cannot laugh while feeling sorry for yourself. Seeing the humor in any situation brings relief and release. Did you hear about the drunk who got a "speeding" ticket after passing out at the wheel of his car? Tragedy, yes. Being able to laugh at the incident in hindsight brings understanding and relief. Our favorite apocryphal joke is about hitting a pig, reporting the accident anonymously and getting a ticket in the mail for $500. And how did they find us, you ask, "the pig squealed."

Shirley set the stage for our approach to her treatment for breast cancer, which included humor and lots of it. On the way in to the operating room for her mastectomy, laying on a gurney in a local community hospital, she said to her surgeon, Phil McWhorter: "Hey, Phil, you ought to charge me half price. I'm pretty small." Courage, strength, fortitude.

A year later, Shirley told the hospital's President & CEO that she was being over charged for her mammogram, that she should get a 50% discount. After all, they only had to take a single x-ray image, not two. What's fair is fair. She left him speechless. It just makes sense to me.

And there was her relationship with her oncologist, Dick Hollister, and his incredible staff. Do you realize that over 95% of cancer treatment takes place in a physician's private office, not in a hospital. If you choose to work in oncology, you know from the get go that at least 50% of your patients will die as a result of their disease. And yet Dick and his staff always provided hope, comfort, and, best of all, laughter and humor.

Dick had made the choice to become a doctor and treat patients with cancer at age 13 according to his mother, at age 11 according to him. He was the perfect match for Shirley, who turned him bright red (fairly easy given his red-head's freckled complexion), when she whipped out her temporary breast prosthesis during his first visit to her hospital room. He was speechless. He knew he had a live one, despite the poor prognosis. Shirley was an interesting and challenging case for a new oncologist in his first few years of practice. Jokes were a staple in his office during the course of our year of treatment. Humor is healing to body, mind, and spirit.

Cry

Real men cry. Real men feel. A good cry is cleansing for the heart, mind and soul. When Shirley's mother and I went home after taking Alison to school, she and I held on to each other for dear life and wept, inconsolably. We each needed to let out the pent-up feelings of anger, helplessness and fear. She feared the loss of a child, her eldest, and her only daughter. I feared the loss of my bride, my partner, my lover, the mother of my one and only child, Alison, who was then just 3 years old. I feared becoming a single parent. How could I, a man, possibly raise a girl, bring her through the formative years and adolescence into adulthood? Was I going to have to date again to find a mother for my daughter, oh, what a wretched, frightening thought.

During the first days after surgery, then over the weeks and on into months, I often found myself alone in the car, driving home, heading to work, whatever. I would be overcome by fear, which was really a lack of faith. Fear and faith cannot co-exist. When emotions hit full blast, I found myself sobbing uncontrollably, tears running down my face, sobs racking my body.

But are there not positive images of men facing loss and pain? The classic Frenchman with tears streaming down his face when the Nazis occupied Paris. Do not men in battle cry when a comrade falls. Crying releases your pent up emotions: anger, fear, sadness, pain, and denial. A safety valve, a mini volcano releasing the pressures from deep within your soul and being. Cry. You feel. You are human and graced. Hug a friend and cry on his or her shoulder. That hug lends strength and comfort.

Follow her lead

Your partner, your bride, knows how she can best deal with her breast cancer. In Shirley's case, she opted for minimal information from day one. She chose to rely on Dick Hollister and Joe Murphy to let her know how she was doing in the simplest of ways. Good or bad blood count, for example, not the numbers, not analysis.

There is no "right" way or "wrong" way. It is her way, her journey, her path. Some patients with cancer try to become oncologists in a heartbeat, reading, reading, and reading more medical literature. Seeking out more and more information, perhaps seeking second, third and fourth opinions. Others may rely on their physician, a man or woman dedicated to healing and life, to be their coach and guide them through the process. Whatever path you choose is the right path for you.

Shirley was the Joe Friday of cancer patients, asking for the facts, nothing but the facts. And keep it short and simple. Shirley did not feel a need to hear or be given all the numbers from her ongoing testing, retesting and testing again. She choose to rely on her physicians, particularly Dick Hollister and Phil McWhorter and their staff, to keep her current with the simplest of terms. Was a blood count good or bad, for example? She did not need or want to hear the numbers. She did not want to analyze her situation. We knew, she knew, that she was "playing for all the marbles," so the outcome was critical, not the steps in the process of survival.

Other women may opt to become overnight medical students or aspiring physicians, trying to learn in an instant what a physician has studied and absorbed over eight years or more. For Shirley and for me, despite my being a clinical social worker and a "health care professional," simple was best. A sound physician-patient relationship is built on mutual respect and trust. It enhances your healing. Trust the coach and run the play.

Being there

Your partner, your wife to whom you have pledged a lifetime commitment, needs to know you are there. She needs a feeling of security. She wants to know that you meant what you said about being together in sickness and in health. Women need, want, and deserve a feeling of security. You are responsible for letting her know and feel that you'll be with her today, tomorrow and forever.

Here we are today, 27 years of marriage later. It was less than easy, but has been steady, up hill, growing, maturing and becoming what God had intended, including being a loving and faithful husband. Foreign territory to a child of the 60's, but sweeter and sweeter as the years went by. It was only through this long, often painful, process that I fully understood the meaning of marriage vows, the sacred nature of a marriage and its importance as the cornerstone, the indispensable and fundamental foundation of civilization as we know it

I love you, not your breasts

Despite our nation's growing obesity, we are a breast and body image fixated society, from Betty Grable pinups in World War II, Marilyn Monroe and Jane Mansfield in the 1950's and 1960's to Salma Hayek and Pamela Anderson today. Men talk about being "leg men" or "breast men" with bravado and sophomoric stupidity, as if large breasts or great legs has anything at all to do with being a woman, or a lifetime companion, or a long-term, intimate lover.

Now, don't get me wrong. I still like to look at and admire beautiful women from the gorgeous 76-year-old former model in a smoking cessation class in 1982 to the stars and women around me. However, it is my bride, my lover, and my lifetime partner who is my sexual and sensual interest today. Your bride, your lover, needs to know that you love who she is, not what type of body she has or the size of her breasts.

Shirley is as beautiful and sexy today as she was on our first date, if not more so. Our love making then and today was not and is not hampered by her having one breast instead of two. Rather, it enriches our intimacy. When we make love, she completes me, makes me whole and alive. God created a matching set that fits together nicely. Your bride needs reassurance in the face of an assault on her femininity and sense of womanhood. She needs to know by what you say and what you do that this set of circumstances is not the end of your sex life, but rather a new, sometimes frightening, and exciting sex life with heightened sensitivity and caring.

Go to her appointments

Go to the multitude of appointments with your wife, your partner, as much as you can, holding her hand literally and figuratively. In 1982, I had the luxury of relative independence on my job as the CEO of a community health and wellness center. I built my professional and community calendar around Shirley's treatment schedule. I went with Shirley to virtually every physician visit, every chemotherapy appointment. I felt a bit guilty about sitting in the waiting room, not going into the exam room with her for the actual treatments. Perhaps a bit of a wimp or squeamish, but I was with her in mind, body and spirit every step of the way. If it were possible, I would have taken it for her, traded places with her.

It is not what you do when you accompany her to treatment, but rather the act itself that speaks volumes to her. It also gives you some sense of empowerment. You are more than a helpless spectator cursing the damned disease. You have joined the battle. You are helping wrest control from the cancer along with your wife, your family and friends, your treatment team and all of the support system around you.

There is also a practical side. Hearing a diagnosis of cancer overwhelms the senses. Doctors try to help you understand, but their daily jargon, the language of medicine, might as well be classical Greek or Latin. With two of you there, there are two sets of ears to hear what is said. There are two mouths to ask questions. This helps avoid the tendency to hear what you want to hear. Being with her each time will reassure her, help her overcome, and make you feel good about yourself. She'll love you for it.

Let her know you're there for the long haul

Remove any fear of abandonment. It is reported that 7 of 10 husbands leave and divorce after their wife is diagnosed and treated for breast cancer. Not very good for we men, however, the same rate of breakup is true for almost any trauma in a couple's life, such as a child with severe disabilities, a handicapping condition, etc. If a marriage relationship is weak, not well grounded, it can be torn asunder. Conversely, a basically solid relationship will become better getting through adversity like this.

We as a culture are experiencing a 60% divorce rate with or without trauma as a precipitating "cause." We now read about young people having "starter marriages" as a prelude to or preparation for a "real" marriage. Whatever happened to "in sickness and in health" or "til death us do part." Be a real man. Love her. Reassure her. Remember the love and the friendship that brought you together. Stay with her. Grow with her. Let her complete you as she did before cancer struck. Your wedding vows are sacred. They are meant for a lifetime.

When the dust settles after this battle, a real man is still standing together with his soul mate, his lover, his bride, the mother of his children.

Help with your child or children

Shirley and I were blessed with one child, our daughter, Alison, who was three years old when we started Shirley's treatment. Dick Hollister, her oncologist, gave us a choice following her surgery: the option of having more children or aggressive treatment that might save Shirley's life, a long shot at best, but a remote possibility. Our decision, our option for life, was instantaneous.

Raising Alison, being her mother, was Shirley's passionate mission. It was her reason for living and surviving, for beating her cancer. Her only major regret or concern was whether she would live to see Alison grow up, become a woman, pursue her dreams, marry, and, God willing, make her a grandmother. There is simply no joy comparable to being a parent, whether a mother or a father. No happiness is greater than being with your child and experiencing their growth.

Shirley was an accomplished and talented elementary school teacher. She might have sought full time employment, but cancer changed her course and our course. She worked part time instead in elementary school and early childhood education to enable her to be home for Alison. She was for all intents and purposes a full-time Mom, the noblest and most difficult of career choices. Perhaps an economic squeeze that allowed Shirley to live her dream and be a real Mom. If you meet Alison, you'll know she made the right choice.

Your children need both of you. Depending on their age, they may or may not really understand what is happening, or share your anxiety and fears. They will know that something is amiss. They need you both. And she will need you to take over more and more as chemotherapy or radiation take their toll, making her tired and sick, taking away her energy and leaving her in need of rest.

She is a warrior doing battle. To win ultimate victory, let her husband (what a marvelous word) her strength and resources. She will do what she can. She will want to be involved. But you need to step in seamlessly when she needs down time. Can you give a greater gift?

Eat your broccoli

When you read anything about breast cancer and nutrition, or other cancers and nutrition, you read about low fat diets and eating cruciferous vegetables. A low fat diet, for example, can slow down prostate cancer. At the top of the list of vegetables most frequently mentioned is broccoli. At the time of Shirley's treatment, Alison loved broccoli and would eat no other vegetable, so we ate broccoli with dinner literally every night for the whole year of treatment. The first President Bush may not have eaten his broccoli, but it was good for us.

It is not beyond the realm of possibility that daily consumption of broccoli enhanced treatment and contributed in some way to Shirley's survival. She suggested just that to her oncologist half jokingly and half seriously. He just shrugged his shoulders, acknowledging that we don't know. He is as surprised at her survival as we are joyful. Perhaps the daily broccoli regimen helped in some unknown way.

Cook a meal

Shirley has always been a great cook, whether making a fancy meal or emptying the refrigerator of all leftovers for a delicious soup. But now is the time to give her a break. You prepare meals from start to finish: shopping, preparing, cooking, serving and especially cleaning up afterwards. That means the whole job, so once again she saves her strength and energy for the important work at hand.

Men are supposed to be the world's greatest chefs, so be one. Bring out your creative and nurturing side, figuratively and literally. Develop a new talent or build on an old one. Out of practice because she's such a good cook, now's the time to plunge back in. Develop your talent. Life is much more enjoyable being a Renaissance man, a multi-talented person using both your right and left-brain.

And she may want simple things, as not all food appeals during the course of chemotherapy treatment. Bon appetit.

Remember pregnancy cravings?
They're back.

Odd, but true, if you've been through pregnancy with your wife, you've had preparation for some of the rigors and nuances of treatment for breast cancer, whether surgery, chemotherapy, hormone therapy, radiation therapy or a combination of all of these. In Shirley's case, following her modified radical mastectomy, we had six months of chemotherapy and hormone therapy, then six weeks of daily radiation therapy, followed by another six months of chemotherapy. A long year for both of us. She was the one getting zapped (as she called it at the time), but we were experiencing treatment.

Shirley applied a lesson from pregnancy to her approach to chemotherapy. When she was pregnant with our daughter, Alison, a friend told her that not all women have severe morning sickness. That knowledge or suggestion led her to a pregnancy with relatively little or mild morning sickness. Mind over matter? The power of self-talk?

Shirley understood in her soul that each of us is unique. Each of us reacts in our own unique manner to chemotherapy. One size does not fit all. As a result, her experience with her very aggressive treatment regimen was relatively mild, at least when compared with horror stories about chemo. She did have her moments, but under-stood she was getting closer each time to the end of treatment and staying alive.

The other parallel to pregnancy was food cravings. I would often be asked to pick up Chocolate Chocolate Hagen-Dazs ice cream, or some other food or beverage she was craving. This ran the gamut from pretzel sticks as a munchie to eating peppermint candy to get rid of the metallic taste left by her chemo treatment. All of this, of course, meant that I was often the family shopper, picking up the groceries, a task that long since was reclaimed by Shirley.

Be available by phone

Have a cell phone and use it. Carry it with you and do not turn it off or miss a call to be polite to others. Cell phone courtesy and etiquette may be an oxymoron these days, but you are not in a position to practice them. This is your wife, your lifetime partner we're talking about. Unless you're getting a direct call from God himself, no one and nothing is more important in your life. Sound vertical alignment calls for God, you, family, country and then everything else. She is your family.

If she needs you, or just wants a few words with you, all else can wait. And will wait. And, once again, need I remind you this is your wife's life we're talking about?

Shirley and I today use a technology that allows us to keep in touch wherever we are. It will search us out until it finds us at one of multiple phones in its memory. Your wife just needs a little of your time, a few words of support, an ability to know that you are there. Her sense of well-being, her ability to cure herself, is enhanced with your providing a sense of security. You are a lifeline. A phone is her link to that lifeline.

She is not an invalid

Your wife or partner is not fragile. She won't break. Treatment can be grueling and tiring, but you both need to live your life as fully as possible. Continue to enjoy what you enjoy individually and as a couple, particularly the latter. One of our best friends and an inspiration for many jogged to her chemotherapy appointments when battling a recurrence of breast cancer. It is called zest for living, being in the now.

Let your bride do anything she is up to trying. In Shirley's case over the course of her year of treatment, that included walks at Greenwich Point, skiing, putting up with some golf with me, puttering with some flowers, and even on occasion agreeing to go sailing with me. You need to take your cues from her. She knows what she can do, or how tired she may be feeling, whether it's a good day or not. When she's ready, encourage her without pushing her. Get out when she's ready.

As I reflect, it was important for Shirley and I to live life fully as a couple and as a family with Alison. We knew our time together here might be very short and we wanted to live our life together fully. We did not anticipate the length of life we've been blessed with together. Shirley is a miracle and so is your wife or partner, no matter what the ultimate outcome.

Take over on chemotherapy nights

In Shirley's case, nothing happened the first time she had chemotherapy. That's when she and I went home together after her treatment at Dick Hollister's office. We sat in the living room of our rented home and waited and watched for something, anything, to happen. Needless to say, nothing occurred. It is the build up of toxins over time that will leave her feeling like she's been hit by the proverbial Mack truck or has a severe case of flu. Over time, she will become very tired, exhausted and whipped. You need to plan ahead and expect to fill in on everything those days.

It is important to remember that each patient's treatment is individualized for her individual case. And each patient will experience her chemotherapy differently. You need to be prepared to step in and take care of all of your children's needs for at least a day or two. You need to be prepared for her being sick by having an ample supply of ginger ale, saltines and peppermint candies. She may also want to be left alone, whether throwing up, or resting quietly in a darkened room. Just go with the flow.

The image that got us through chemotherapy was Louise Crisafi's making an analogy to the then popular video game, Pac Man. She said to imagine that the chemotherapy drugs were running around Shirley's system gobbling up the cancer cells. It was a great image to visualize and believe in.

Do *not* buy her a scarf or head covering

I blew this one big time. I trusted my intuition or my need to cope. I sought out and bought a couple of head coverings before Shirley's hair fell out. Being a former Boy Scout, I was trying to "be prepared" ahead of time. That was perhaps my biggest mistake. As a man, whether you're bald or not, need to understand the real, tangible and symbolic importance of your bride's hair. It is her mane, another visible sign of her femininity. Losing it is just one more assault after the loss of a breast. It has tremendous impact on her feelings of self worth and being a woman.

Michael was Shirley's hairdresser in 1982. Both Michael and Shirley assured Dick Hollister, her oncologist, and me that she was NOT going to lose her hair and end up bald. Dick and I both believed they were wrong, that they shared a fantasy that was not to be. Shirley and Michael knew better. They were right. Shirley's hair thinned, but it did not depart. I was in the doghouse and the headscarf was in the attic, never to be seen or used.

Unlike Robert Young in the 1950's television series *Father Knows Best*, father or husband does not always know best, particularly when it comes to a woman's needs. It is critical that we take our clues from our partner. If she wants to get a wig or a scarf, she'll know when it's time.

And this is not something you can pick out for her.

Learn from prostitutes.

Do I have your attention? Sex sells. I am not suggesting that you employ their services. Your best sex is found at home with your lifetime partner. Period.

Shirley found a new gynecologist as she went through treatment, Ed Jacobson, a warm man, the kind of physician whose presence and demeanor is comforting and reassuring by nature. He enriched our lives, specifically our sex lives, by suggesting we try jellies and creams to make intercourse easier and more comfortable after you partner has been through menopause, whether naturally, or, as in Shirley's case, as a result of chemotherapy and hormone therapy. Early menopause was induced at age 37. In explaining their use to Shirley during an office visit, he described it as "the stuff used by prostitutes in Stamford." Sounded like good advice to her and to me. And, by the way, it does work.

There is sex after mastectomy, wonderful, beautiful, glorious sex. And, in the beginning, it can be simultaneously exquisite and painful. There is nothing that can quite prepare a man for making love, and having intercourse, with the love of his life who he fears losing. The threat hung over our heads and was part of our thoughts for days, months and years. Shirley would be embarrassed were I to say any more about our sex life. It is intimate.

Another lesson from prostitutes

Women of the evening, sex workers as they're know in Nevada or members of the world's oldest profession, do know the best sources of wigs for a woman who loses her hair. You as a husband and partner need to understand intellectually and emotionally that whatever wig she finds, she is not getting it to wear after her hair grows back in. It is not beautiful. It is a temporary, and sometimes devastating, accommodation to the reality she is facing. She wants to look her best, but she does not want suggestions or inferences that it will be around for the long term.

My sister, Margaret, who completed breast cancer treatment, did not want to hear comments about her new growth of hair or show it until it was really back. And she points out that the "coming out" can be difficult. Again, a parallel to pregnancy: just as well meaning friends and strangers want to touch your belly when you're pregnant, the same friends will reach out to touch your new growth. This is a difficult, complex and emotional issue. Wigs work and have a function, but being able to get rid of them is a sign of recovery, of being able to move on with life.

Pray

We've heard often that there are no atheists in foxholes. Well, you're now in a foxhole. There is a war to be won on the home front. If you didn't pray before, there's no better time to learn. It is as simple as thinking or talking to a friend. God is here. He will hear you.

Shirley and I have had our "fair share" of challenges from my congenital birth defect that left me with a leaky aortic valve, starting on a life-long, day at a time path of recovery from alcoholism just 361 days after we were married. Alison had a "congenital dislocated hip" discovered during a routine pediatric check-up at age 6 months. This resulted in her having a week in traction in a small rural hospital, where she had been born via Cesarean, through "minor" surgery (always an oxymoron, since no surgery is minor), and followed by 2 months in a body cast and 10 months in a body brace.

A few years after Shirley's treatment, I had a stubborn, difficult to diagnose pain in my side. After months of tests, I was told I had a "hot" rib and would need to have a biopsy performed by a thoracic surgeon. Was it cancer? Another malignancy in the family? No, but my 10th rib on the right side was removed. A rather rare case of fibromyalgia, a benign, but dangerous cartilage-like growth. It turned out to be good "practice" several years later when I had aortic valve replacement surgery at Yale-New Haven Hospital. Again, a chest tube, wires and lots of other tubes in various parts of my body. I now tick like the crocodile in Peter Pan.

The point is that God does not give us more than we can handle, although we may object to some his character building. Ed Vicinanza, a friend and mentor, has reinforced my understanding of what is truly important in life, what he calls our vertical alignment, placing God first followed by family, work or business and the rest of our life interests.

Belief helps. Faith is belief turned into action. Living itself is an act of faith. Raising a child is faith. Trusting your physician is faith. Asking prayer groups in your community or elsewhere to include you or a loved one in their prayers is an act of faith. Shirley has lived her life faithfully. Her namesake, the late Aunt Shirley Durgin, gave her a subscription to *Daily Word* for devotions and meditations. She has been reading those and others for years. Her survival has been a miracle. It has also been an act of faith and dogged determination on her part.

She is your trophy wife

You need to understand that your bride, your wife, the woman you promised to cherish, the love of your life and your best friend is also the answer to your caricature male mid-life crisis. The answer is not a young intern wearing a thong who's young enough to be your daughter. It is not a young bimbo or young colleague with whom to start your next marriage, or your next family. It is not a sports car, a speedboat or a new set of golf clubs. It is your wife.

I encountered this attitude and understanding observing the marriage of Joe and Shirley Robinson, two "adolescents in love" after more than 40 years of marriage. Rather than have a midlife crisis alternative relationship, whether sexual or emotional, how about a fling with your wife. Take her away for a comfy weekend at a romantic bed and breakfast. In our case, it can be some quiet time together in the Berkshires. Or perhaps a Broadway show, or a good movie and an after show dessert. Fall in love. Stay in love. Be in love.

Use complementary, integrative or alternative medicine

Shirley and I believe in the miracle that is modern medicine, whether that is the multiple therapies that saved her life or the artificial valve in my heart. We also know that modern medicine has at times thrown out the baby with the bath water. A placebo effect, the impact of a physician's belief that you would get better on your own belief, has been show to have a positive effect. It is not "scientific" these days, so it is a pejorative term. We seem to have lost sight of the fact that medicine remains even today 2% science and 98% art.

When I first saw a cardiologist at Yale in preparation for valve replacement surgery, he set aside the piles of medical records and reports to see, feel and hear using the simplest tools of trade: his hands, his ears and a stethoscope. After a few minutes of listening, thumping on my chest, and hands on touching, he rated me a 3 on a scale of 1 to 4. This meant 75% of the blood being pumped out through my aorta was leaking back into the heart, not a very comforting image. He then picked up the volumes of medical records, flipped through and confirmed his assessment. Healing arts are real. I was privileged to have a new artificial valve put in my heart on August 28, 1991. However, it was my faith and the faith and support of those around me that gave me the calm assurance needed to survive and thrive.

You and your wife should feel free to use Eastern and other holistic modalities to complement your Western medical treatment. Vitamins and supplements, for example, are a routine part of medical practice in Germany and their knowledge is spreading to the United States. When Shirley asked, a physician supported her decision to spread liquid Vitamin E on the portion of her chest receiving radiation in order to prevent radiation burns. It worked. She came through her six weeks of daily radiation treatment with flying colors and little radiation burn. The irony is that the physician asked her not to tell others of his suggestion, as they might think him a "kook" or outside the mainstream for supporting its use. One caution, talk openly and fully with your physician about other treatments, particularly herbs or vitamins, to be sure there are no contraindications. This is comparable to avoiding potentially dangerous or even lethal mixing of prescription medications.

A tai chi instructor is an advocate of tai chi as a complement to traditional therapies, including rehabilitation patients. In her own case as a patient with cancer, she found her tai chi helpful in getting her through chemotherapy more easily.

Find something that works for you. There are innumerable complements or enhancements to your medical care that have a beneficial effect on body, mind and spirit. They include: prayer and meditation, prayer groups, vitamins and herbs, yoga, tai chi, acupuncture, reiki therapy, feng shui, energy healing, morning pages, support groups. Each has something to offer. Let your physician know what you are doing, but do not expect him or her to understand, know about and/or approve of most modalities.

Use the serenity prayer

God, grant me the serenity to accept the things I cannot change, courage to change the things I can, and the wisdom to know the difference.

I first heard of this prayer from my mother in the last few years of her all too short life (she died at 60). It meant nothing other than I vaguely understood it comforted her. And then I heard it, spoke it, and began to apply it in my own life.

We could not change Shirley's diagnosis, nor could we be responsible for the responses of friends, family and colleagues. One or two "friends" disappeared off the face of the earth unable to be near illness. Most friends jumped in to help and support us in any way possible. In each instance, the choice was theirs to make, not ours. In retrospect and seeing the results, perhaps we did have the courage required to change the prognosis. Shirley's being here today, healthy and whole, speaks volumes for faith and prayer and overcoming unbeatable odds. Facts don't count. People do. God does.
Shirley and I both knew we could work on us, on our acceptance of the situation or circumstances we faced. We could determine to win the war against this insidious disease with Shirley herself leading and inspiring us in battle after battle, day by day overcoming, surviving and thriving.

Lemonade from lemons

When life gives you lemons, make lemonade. See the silver lining. You are not a Pollyanna to find something exquisite, profound and meaningful in facing cancer, facing death and facing loss. Can you imagine yourself in the shoes or the psyche of a person with cancer? Or as the husband, lover and lifetime partner of a woman with breast cancer? Can you understand deep in your soul what intimacy is like, sexual and otherwise, when all your senses are stretched and heightened by the knowledge you're making love to a woman you could lose?

You find joy to the point of pain. You discover a profound sense of being one with each other, and yet there is awareness that it could be fleeting and transitory. Reality may break in and shatter the moment, but you persevere. I have often said in the years since "our" treatment for Shirley's breast cancer that a good marriage, or a solid relationship, will not only get through the trauma of breast cancer, the marriage will be strengthened and be the better for it. Go figure.

Anger

Let your anger out. Shirley was very little on the "why me" or "poor me" approach to her disease and her treatment. She was angry about the thought of not seeing Alison grow up. She knew she had a battle to fight and a war to win. It didn't matter why. What did matter were survival, good health, and living into our dotage. Or at least until Alison grew up, went through college and perhaps started a family along with pursuing her dreams.

In other words, Shirley's passion, her overriding concern, was to be a mother to her child, her only child. The one and only thought that brought her to venting her anger was the possibility of not seeing Alison grow up. Shirley vented her rage in our kitchen sink. She threw old glasses into the sink, smashing them one by one, and having a good cry. Very satisfying. Quite cathartic. My preference was pounding the steering wheel while driving the car and sobbing. It's OK.

The point is that anger is OK, as long as it doesn't cripple you. Living life fully and passionately relieves the anger.

One Day At A Time

Shirley and I quit smoking on October 28, 1976 thanks to an eight-week commercial smoking cessation program. One of the key lessons learned then and reapplied less than a year later, when starting my lifelong recovery from alcoholism, was learning to live a day at a time. We did not have to think about never, ever, never having another cigarette. Rather, it was just for 15 minutes after a meal or while driving the car, and then it became not smoking today and today only. Having started sneaking cigarettes at age 11 and smoking 2-3 packs a day, I was the most surprised when I stopped.

Shirley and I had learned that lesson together, so it was natural to use it with her, and our, battle against her cancer. It was a critical part of her and our recovery. We got through the visit with her new surgeon, Phil McWhorter, which confirmed the need for a breast biopsy. We got through making a choice between one-step or two-step biopsy and surgery for removal of her breast. We got through knowing and accepting that Alison was to be our only child. What a blessing she was and is to this day. We got through the first chemo treatment, and the second, and the third, and the fourth and on through a long, grueling year. We went through treatment a day at a time, or ate the elephant one bite at a time.

Avoid doom and gloom

You need optimism and positive thinking. You need to surround yourself with survivors and winners. You know who they are. You see it in their aura, their smile, and their attitudes. There is an inner strength that radiates from these people, whether it is your wife's Reach to Recovery volunteer, another member of a recovery program or an artist sharing his or her work.

What you don't need or want is "friends," family or colleagues who suck out all of the light when they enter a room. These are the "woe is me, oh, ain't it awful" types. Their cup is always half empty at best, usually seen as worse, no matter what the situation or circumstances. This is the person who still asks me "How's Shirley?" and thinks I'll be reporting her demise or a recurrence of her cancer.

I fill my heart and soul with positive by reading daily: Proverbs in the morning, plus positive mental attitude books before going to sleep at night. You can't read Og Mandino's "Memo From God" at the end of *The Greatest Miracle in the World* without gaining a profound understanding of what a gift our physical being is. A reading and application of the principles and techniques in Julia Cameron's *The Artist's Way* provides insight and understanding of synchronicity and of God's abundance, which is ours for the asking.

You and your bride need to be up. You need to believe. Latch on to the optimists and the faithful around you. Develop a positive mental attitude and spirit. Keep the faith.

Have fun

No matter what the prognosis, she is not dead, nor are you. You both need to live. You need to be joyful. You need to allow yourself to have fun. Our good friend and a saint here on earth, Louise Crisafi, modeled this for us when fighting an ultimately losing battle with a virulent recurrence of breast cancer. She and her husband, Bart, who was and is my cardiologist, took 2-3 trips a year to Italy. They found the real Italy of their ancestors, the joyful places to be one with each other and their ancestry. Louise and Bart took their last trip together the week before she died. They had a wonderful Bermuda vacation, came home to a weekend with family, and her passing on Monday in a local hospital. She set the standard for being more and over-coming.

Treat yourselves in large ways and small. Take her out to dinner, preferably a quiet, romantic ambience. Send her flowers for no reason. Go to a movie and munch on popcorn. See a play or a concert. Perhaps a ball game. Be a true romantic on Valentine's Day. I hit a home run this year when I "snuck out" at 3am in the morning to buy two valentine cards, a helium balloon and flowers. It was one of the few times I've been able to surprise Shirley.

There is more to your life than being a patient with cancer or being the husband of a woman with cancer. You are all the rest that is you, too. Be those parts. Live those activities. Get your mind off the cancer by keeping the rest of your life full of its daily blessings.

She is not damaged goods

A man attending a prostate cancer support group expressed concern about being "damaged goods" following prostate cancer treatment. Your bride is *not* damaged goods with or without breast reconstruction. She remains the woman you fell in love with, the woman you committed to for a lifetime together. Get beyond the inner thoughts never expressed, wondering whether your lovemaking was altered forever. You, too, may miss her breast, as it has brought you both pleasure in the past. Whether or not to have breast reconstruction is a personal choice, her choice. Shirley chose not to do so, in part I believe to avoid furthering tampering with and "awakening" any missed cancer cells.

Now is the time to live your life to its fullest together. Cleave to her. Hold her. Love her. Smell her. Taste her. Smile with her. Laugh with her. Cry with her. Get angry with her. Yes, you still have "negative" feelings and emotions. You are still human beings in the ebb and flow of a love relationship that is more intense than most of those around you. You'll both survive and thrive if you stay together.

Chivalry is not dead

An occasional actor, I have had just two roles that I loved playing: Sir Lancelot during our senior high school class production of A Connecticut Yankee in King Arthur's Court and the fumbly, bumbly King and loving father in Thurber's Many Moons. Perhaps both were a hangover from my reading over and over the story of King Arthur and the story of Robin Hood.

Knights in shining armor are welcome by women today, as are gentlemen and gentle men. Chivalrous is synonymous with manful-ness and manliness. It is part of our nature. It is more than OK to hold open a door, pull out a chair and do all of the other "little things" that say you respect and admire her. You are subordinating yourself to her. And please, don't forget to take off your hat, or inverted baseball cap (God, help us) when you're indoors. Hats off. Bring her flowers when she's not expecting them. Or chocolate, even when she protests about her diet.

You might say I am a traditionalist. So be it. Your bride will love you for it and you'll feel special by making her feel special. Join the Round Table! Restore Camelot.

Read Proverbs

If you could have just one guide on living life, perhaps the best self-help guide in the history of mankind, other than the Holy Bible itself, is Proverbs 1-31. One of the men who has had the most significant impact on my faith and spiritual life, as well as my commitment to family and dreams, is Ed Vicinanza, a mentor, friend and spiritual teacher. He leads and teaches others by example.

I rediscovered my own faith in 1977. It was Ed who advised me to use Proverbs 1-31 as a form of daily meditation. It is ordered, logical, deep and measurable. Your book mark will tell you daily whether or not you are being consistent, whether or not you are truly committed to developing your spiritual life, your wisdom, and your understanding of God's guidance for living.

Like you, I am a human being working on being a spiritual being. Maintaining this daily habit is not as easy or automatic as brushing teeth or taking a shower. It is like the discipline needed to succeed at anything, whether that is exercising daily, building a business, organizing daily life or whatever. Proverbs requires a daily commitment to early morning devotional reading. You might want to supplement Proverbs with other daily meditations of your own choosing.

The key is to keep at it. You will find wisdom, guidance and faith, a direction for your life and living that is priceless. Keep the faith.

Read Psalms for Health & Healing

It is part of the synergy in my life and the universe that I attended a talk by Rabbi Charles P. Rabinowitz on prayer for health and healing in the "Second Hour" at First Congregational Church in Old Greenwich, Connecticut. I was transfixed and enthralled, as he went through ten Psalms he recommended as a guide for prayer and meditation for maintaining health or battling illness and disease.

The ten Psalms offer a comprehensive remedy or general healing and include Psalms 16, 32, 41, 42, 59, 77, 90, 105, 137 and 150. Psalm 16 offers hope and asks for God's direction in our lives, while Psalm 32 utilizes anticipatory hope of being recovered. Psalm 41 meditates on suffering, which is experienced by each of us, while Psalm 42 speaks of the soul's anguish and reliance on faith as we encounter illness. Psalm 59 faces tragedy and despair transforming it into gratitude and thanksgiving. Psalm 77 helps us understand that God is with us through our life journey, no matter how dark, no matter what we face. Psalm 90 reflects on the challenges of daily living and maintaining a semblance of normalcy in the midst of our encounters with cancer, loss of work, loss of relationship or any of the other myriad bumps in the road. Psalm 105 offers two paths to healing and Psalm 137 expresses our pain, our yearning to return to a

Jerusalem state of mind and physical being. Psalm 150 brings closure and praises God with the very gift that God gave us to keep us alive, our breath.

These ten psalms together provide a unique calming of the spirit, a necessary step on the path to healing. By the end of the talk, I knew we were meant to meet each other, that I could incorporate these ten Psalms in my morning meditations, thereby adding to my contact with God, enhancing my understanding of God's will. It is not coincidence that Rabbi Rabbinowitz's wife was a recent breast cancer survivor. The message was there. Again, it is a matter of discipline. After you finish your Proverb of the day, just turn to the Psalm of the day. You can read each three times a month, once every ten days.

Be trustworthy

Fidelity, honor, trust. Old fashioned ideals? Pie in the sky? Not realistic? Missing out? No one else is? Balm for mid-life crisis makes it necessary? I just don't accept the direction we've headed. Fidelity to your bride, your life's partner, is a sacred obligation and responsibility. It is also a gift. You are getting beyond the human drives and instincts to a spiritual level of intimacy and relationship that transcends and enhances your life.

You honor your wife by being faithful. During the course of treatment for breast cancer, this act of being faithful, the choices made day in and day out, support your partner, help make her whole, let her know you love her. Can you imagine the impact of an extramarital affair on the self image and sense of worth of your partner, as your sexual partner, were you to stray.

Adultery is unconscionable at any time in any marriage. It is even more despicable when your partner has been through removal of a breast, the rigors of chemotherapy and hormone therapy, the blasts of radiation treatment.
Are you a man in the image of God, or are you a swine? Trust in a marriage of necessity must be one hundred percent. You cannot be a little unfaithful.

Be a good listener

Your wife, your partner, takes her cue from whether or not you are listening to her. As she goes through treatment, it is time for you to be there for her and not be distracted. Put the paper down. Turn off the game on TV. She needs your attention. She needs to communicate in a manner that supports her recovery and cure.

You have read about people who simply listen to a friend or colleague, perhaps throw in a few "uh huhs," say few if any words, and are deemed great communicators. Now is the time to practice that art. Tune in. Listen with your heart. Listen with your mind. Listen with your soul. Try to understand her and her needs. That is paramount as you face the battle together.

Listening is the best form of communication.

Take her to treatments

I will never forget sitting in Phil McWhorter's office and understanding deep in my soul, that based on his physical examination of Shirley's right breast, we were undoubtedly facing a diagnosis of breast cancer. A biopsy could confirm it, but it was almost certain. Now, at the time, I had been "in the health care industry" for ten years. I was a "professional," educated to be a clinical social worker. In my work, including talks on breast cancer and other diseases, I stressed the importance of a positive, optimistic outlook, that a cancer diagnosis was not a death sentence. But, as a human being, as a father of a 3-year-old daughter, as a husband of five years, I felt Shirley's diagnosis as if it were a death sentence. Cancer, the BIG C. Life was over. All those thoughts and feelings in a moment, but not voicing them or letting them out. Keeping up a positive front so as not to scare her.

When we started treatment, meaning she was getting zapped, poisoned, radiated or how ever else you might describe it, I was along for the ride. I made it a point to drive her to her appointments. I felt a bit cowardly that I stayed in the waiting room during the treatment itself, but at least I was there. It is a comfort and support for her. Equally important, it gives you some sense of control yourself. You feel less helpless. You're no longer just a spectator watching and hoping. You are helping. You are taking action against this insidious disease. She feels better. You feel better. And perhaps you help bring on the cure.

Bring her home if she wants to be home

Most women work because their families need the money. If your wife wants to be at home or wants to be a full time mother to your children, make it happen. There is nothing more important in our lives than raising our children, truly God's blessing in our lives.

When our daughter, Alison, was born, Shirley stayed home on maternity leave, first for six months, then for more. She reluctantly returned to work, teaching kindergarten. She knew immediately that caring for and teaching 25 children for other parents was infinitely less important and less rewarding than being a Mom. She wanted to be there for Alison, raising and loving her as only a Mom can.

We wanted to make ends meet, to have as much money as there was month. And then I moved us to Greenwich to "further my career," take an upwardly mobile position as the CEO of a local health agency. A little more than a year after our relocation, cancer hit our family.

Shirley was facing what appeared to be certain death. Her cancer was widespread. It was an aggressive variety, a virulent form of breast cancer. She wanted to live. She wanted to be here to see Alison go through toddler stage, grade school, adolescence and beyond. She wanted to be at her wedding. She wanted to be a grandmother some day. She instinctively knew this. Facing her mortality, knowing that she might not be here long, Shirley's first and only priority, other than beating the odds and surviving, was to be a Mom to Alison.

Her choice and ultimately our choice was to do without, to sacrifice, so that Alison would have a Mom raising her, rather than a low paid day care center worker. No one can love and care for a child like its Mom. Children deserve a mother. Alison deserved Shirley, so we made it work. I honestly don't know how we managed at times, but it worked. And the apple did not fall far from the tree. If you met our daughter, you'd understand the value of having Mom at home. We skimped compared to our two-income friends, but we found riches beyond compare. Bring her home!

What you say

The power is in the word, in your word or words. What you say matters. It effects you, the people around you and everything about you. Particularly powerful are the words you say about yourself, about your condition or circumstances. The principle comes from God himself leading the way. God said "Let there be light, and there was light.

This is the power of positive thinking and the power of the spoken word. If I say and believe I am thin, I will be or will become thin. Shirley was determined to live. She said she was going to survive. She said she was keeping her hair. When asked, I said she was doing great, no matter what the circumstances at that point. If I spoke it into existence, others would follow suit and add in their vision of Shirley surviving. Perhaps a form of communal prayer for healing and health. It works.

Believe in miracles

We read about miracles all the time, day in and day out, week after week, year after year. The expression is a cliché to some, but a matter of truth and profound faith to others.

Your battle, and our battle, with cancer is the same thing. We, you and your bride, must believe that she will survive no matter what the odds. Shirley was facing a prognosis that was bleak to say the least, perhaps a five to ten percent chance of survival.

Shirley's odds were one in ten at best, probably much less. But her belief, her deeply held faith, led her to the understanding that she would be the one of the one in ten who indeed would survive. She was not going to be one of the nine in ten who succumbed to the disease. She simply refused to roll over and die. She refused to concede defeat. If knocked down, she got back up. She was stronger than the cancer ravaging her body. She fought back relying on her God to bring her through.

To this day, we know that Dick Hollister is surprised and amazed that he worked a miracle in treating Shirley. He had no doubt she was going to die, as do at least 50% or more of any oncologist's patients. Shirley has joked with him in recent years about knowing that he didn't expect her to survive, that he is surprised to see her alive and vibrant. It is also true that some when asking "How's Shirley?, ask with the expectation that the other shoe will have dropped, that she has had a recurrence. And yet she is here, alive and well.

Odds of survival are meaningless. You are not an aggregate of the number of cases. You are one person. You are you. You are one case, not many. You need to believe and you need to speak being the survivor. It works.

Bride for life

There can be nothing worse in a marriage relationship than letting it grow stale or dull. I have forever it seems and to this day referred to Shirley as my bride, and this is true today, having been married for more than 26 years. This habit, this way of referring to her, seems like an instinctive reach to keep us young as a couple, to keep the joy and excitement of our romance a part of our lifetime together.

Shirley is my business partner. She is my cheerleader. She is the strong woman behind every successful man. She is the mother of my daughter, Alison, for which I am forever grateful and blessed. And this is all the result of making the plunge, not giving up on lifetime commitment, and marrying the woman matched for me by God.

Shirley completes me. We are one. A lifetime commitment keeps the awe and joy of our first day as husband and wife in the forefront. I do not forget from whence we started. Keep it in your heart and carry it forward.

Pay it forward

Shirley was led through her treatment and recovery by a friend, the late Louise Crisafi, an American Cancer Society Reach to Recovery volunteer. Louise and I worked closely together, she as a volunteer serving on my board of directors and me as staff, so it was natural that both Shirley and I turned to her for support, direction, comfort and understanding. Perhaps most important, we needed her faith, her profound belief in a caring, compassionate Christian God.

Like most Reach to Recovery volunteers, Louise gave Shirley hope, belief that she could beat her cancer. She helped Shirley through the process of choosing between a one-step and a two-step biopsy and surgery. She let me know what I could do to be of help. She visited. She called. She was a presence in our lives, particularly Shirley's.

Shirley wondered what she could do to repay her and Louise's response was to pass it on to another woman in need, to pay it forward as demonstrated so beautifully in the recent movie by that name. Shirley chose 21 years ago, in the era when breast cancer was beginning to come out of the closet, to be public and open about her disease and her treatments. That was a fateful decision that over the years has probably saved a life or two, women who knew her or knew of her finally deciding to have their mammogram and checkup. It also brought and continues to bring countless phone calls from women who need and want to talk it through.

When Louise had a recurrence that ultimately took her life, we confided in each other. She was one of the first "civilians" who learned of my alcoholism and my day-to-day recovery. It was a bond that was felt by both of us. I keep my life by giving it away.

Be passionate about life

I still remember a sparrow sitting on a small branch at Todd's Point in Old Greenwich at 6am on a cool Spring morning. I cannot walk by that spot to this day and not remember. One example of "stop to smell the roses" and be aware of the beautiful world around us. We need that more and more as our lives continue to speed up at a frenetic pace with the advent of cell phones, faxes, e-mail and phone conferencing. See a sunset. Smell the lilacs. Stop to think, to meditate.

Coming close to losing your life is a tough way to learn to appreciate life and living. I hearken back to my childhood, lying on very rich, dark green grass in our back yard on Borthwick Avenue. A long flower bed behind my head and to my left to the end of the yard. Staring at two apple trees above me and a Cherry tree to my right side. And thinking about God, about life. Observing clouds. Wondering how far the universe stretches, as well as what's on the other side. Trying to take in and understand the infinite. And also worrying about my mortality. How would I die? Was there something, anything after this life? What would it be like to die?

Facing death in the here and now brought us up short. We had to reassess. We had to understand and act on what is important, truly important. We need to savor life and all it has to offer. Smell the flowers. Taste the apple. Watch the sun dip into the ocean at Key West. Plunge through a grove of birch and pine trees in 3-4 inches of newly fallen, virgin, powder snow. Be in awe of nesting bald eagles on Turtle Island in Winter Harbor, Maine.

Life is precious. Live it fully. Experience it.

Enjoy the mundane

I have found it very comforting to be normal, whatever that may be, to enjoy the simple things in life. It is every day activities that are the mosaic, not great adventure or celebrity. It is taking a walk together, going to a PTA meeting, having dinner with good friends, watching at Tumble Bugs gymnastics or at a t-ball game. Or washing dishes and using that time for quiet thought.

It is these simple things in life that are the most wonderful. When you face your mortality, you and your bride understand that it is the little things that are important, taking a walk together, holding hands, sharing a meal, going to work, the cat cuddling in your arm. It is not glitz and excitement. Rather, it is the ongoing routines and traditions of life. It is wrapping Christmas presents and sneaking them under the tree. It is holding hands as a family and speaking about what each of us is thankful for. It is being in a room without needing to speak. It is enjoying just being with your family, old and young, each generation.

Chemotherapy

You can find plenty of information on chemotherapy in your physician's office, online now that we have the internet from the National Cancer Institute, the American Cancer Society and scores of other reputable sites. There is plenty of information.

What Shirley and I learned together that chemotherapy, much like any experience, is unique to the person experiencing it. Shirley applied a thought process she learned during her pregnancy carrying Alison. A friend happened to mention that not all women have severe or serious morning sickness. Having been given that thought, Shirley spoke it and thought it into reality. She did not experience much morning sickness and queasiness.

A friend told her the same thing about chemotherapy. First, each patient has an individualized or customized regimen depending on the nature of their tumor, its stage and other factors. Not everyone gets sick and throws up, or at least not all the time. Shirley passes this knowledge on often. We did, of course, go home after her first treatment, sat in the living room and waited for something, anything to happen. Nothing did.

What we learned over time was that Shirley would lose a day or so after each treatment, as the toxins built up in her system and lowered her immune system defenses. She knew she would be tired and need to take it easy. Alison and I knew we were on our own, or were doing what we could to help and support her.

The most important lesson was the visualization given to us by Louise. She suggested that we think of the chemo as a form of Pac Man, who was running around her system eating up ALL of the cancer cells. He was cleansing her system. Could you think of a more perfect visual for healing.

Radiation Therapy

Can you get used to the idea that many of the treatments being given to the love of your life are avoided by those who are healthy? When we have a simple dental x-ray, we are used to the weight of a heavy lead shield on our chest. Or the x-ray technician stepping out of the room while he zaps you with a chest x-ray.

Now, at some point in the course of treatment, radiation therapy may become the treatment of choice or one additional treatment that might possibly add to her chances of survival. One physician described the various treatments, and whether or not to choose them, as the combination belt and suspenders approach to treatment.

As planned, Shirley under went radiation therapy five days a week for six weeks following her first six months of chemotherapy: Precise computerized radiation treatment plans were relatively new in 1983, so we were relying on the "old fashioned" shotgun approach to radiation therapy. My unspoken fear was that it could be a fatal judgement call, but I also knew we had left some of the tumor in her chest wall. I prayed that we were killing off as many of the remaining critters as possible, taking the risk of "collateral damage," but giving Shirley her best chance for life and longevity.

Your wife will make a choice based on what's right for her in consultation with her oncologist, the quarterback and coach of her cancer team, and perhaps with the advice of an active tumor board at your community hospital cancer center. Six to eight heads are always better than one and bring together a necessary balance in perspectives on treatment options and direction.

Shirley was her own best advocate. She was prepared for the inevitable tiring and weakening caused over weeks by the daily doses of radiation therapy. She addressed one of her own personal concerns, the likelihood of her chest getting radiation burn in the process. A physician recommended she apply liquid Vitamin E on her chest before each treatment. It worked. There was little or no burn.

Hormone Therapy

Shirley was at the time what we now know was the leading edge of the trend toward diagnosis and treatment of younger and younger women with breast cancer. This is one way in which we had not set out to set a trend, but so be it. Her combination of medications to kill the cancer cells brought on the equivalent of menopause at age 37 and all it entails, e.g., weight gain, hot flashes, dryness, inability to have more children.

We learned together to make adjustments. I take coumadin daily, so I tend to be cold. Shirley has hot flashes and tends to be warm. Some how, we make it all work without freezing me

You are both a miracle

When you reflect on who you are and where you came from, meaning your mother and father, and your grandparents on each side of the family, and your grandparents' parents and on back into the not so distant past, it is hard not to be awed. If you go back just 20 generations, 600 years or so, you and your wife each individually is the net sum of one and half million ancestors. Can you understand and grasp how unique, rare and special that makes each one of you. Snowflakes are unique, so are you and so is she.

One of my favorite writers, Og Mandino, in *The Greatest Miracle in the World*, amplifies this wonder in his classic "Memorandum From God." A piece of that is how unique each one of us is given the number of possible combinations contained in the genes and chromosomes of that single egg and single sperm that united to create you, your wife, me, my wife, our daughter.

The wonder of life and of being grows with each passing day. The medical technology of today is giving us truly incredible glimpses of life in the womb, even now being able to treat a baby in utero. Understand you are helping one of God's miracles to overcome breast cancer and live out her life with you. Keep the faith. Choose health. Choose life.

Synchronicity

We often hear there are no coincidences in life; things happen as they are supposed to, as God designed, or perhaps when we are ready and prepared for what he has to offer. It is not an accident that a good friend opened my eyes to the value of being a writer, which headed me into op ed writing on a small scale, magazine column writing and profuse writing in my career. It is not an accident that one of the few undergraduate courses I worked at and excelled in was with a marvelous professor who taught freshman writing like no other English teacher: discipline and craft. It is not an accident that I was challenged by an acquaintance to write this book, having thought about doing so for years.

What does this have to do with your wife's treatment for breast cancer? Nothing and everything. People will drop out of your life and others will "magically" appear just when you need them. I asked a special friend, a woman 18 years my senior, to be a spiritual mentor just four weeks before Shirley's diagnosis. I had never specifically asked for help like that before then. She was responsible for my understanding and knowing in my gut and my soul that I could get through this, or through anything. She gave me the strength to be strong for Shirley and being a woman, rather than a man as suggested, was the right gender at the right moment.

Trust your instincts.   Be ready for the possibilities. Recognize God working in your life. See the wheels of the universe turning in your direction to ease the way and make things happen.

Thoughtful Gifts

Doing something, virtually anything, truly is the difference. It is the thought behind your gifts and remembrances that counts, not their dollar value. Whether it's her birthday, your anniversary, Valentine's Day or the myriad other opportunities, she will appreciate anything and everything you do without prompting.

No man understands women, nor should we be expected to do so. We do not think, feel or behave the same. However, I do know that Shirley and all women do not mean it when they tell you not to get a present, that "we can't afford," ot "it's not important." Hog wash. Do something for her and do it on time without her prompting.

My best home run that I can put my finger on in our first 26 years of marriage was a combination of flowers, helium balloon and a great card left at the bottom of our stairs for Shirley to find in the morning. A home run! One other home run was buying her a new set of exquisite modern skis (she is an avid and graceful skier who makes it look effortless) for Christmas.

Bottom line, pamper your bride. She deserves it. You might lose her. Better to be in debt financially that to be in debt emotionally, but you need not spend much. Be thoughtful. This is the woman you love, the mother of your children. Remember her all of the time.

Be a romantic. Write love notes. Leave then under her pillow, in a book she's reading, or on the bathroom mirror. Let her know she is the center of your life, whether you have another six months (what I thought) or another thirty years.

Speak Up for Her & for You

Your bride and you need to be comfortable speaking up for her needs during the course of treatment and beyond. A specific example in our case occurred when Shirley started her radiation therapy. Facing the unknown with all the fears that accompany beginning a new therapy, a new modality, another toxic treatment designed to kill cancer cells, and what happened: Shirley was left waiting for an hour for what would be a few minutes of treatment.

Each of you starting treatment or going through treatment understand that additional stress like this is unwanted and unnecessary. And Shirley is an aggressive consumer capable of speaking up for her needs, her rights and her wants. She let her radiologist know that his team's level of care was simply unacceptable and why it was unacceptable. She had just completed her first six months of chemotherapy. This was not a time to handle her in such a cavalier, thoughtless manner.

Bottom line. She stood up for herself. She spoke up. She was not docile. And she never waited again during that entire six weeks of radiation therapy, or in subsequent years when having her annual mammogram.

And what does this have to do with you, her husband. Unlike her being aggressive at a store or haggling over price at a flea market and you being embarrassed, you must be comfortable with her standing up for what she needs. Indeed, you might have to do that for her at times during the course of treatment.

Good Patient, Bad Patient

Different strokes for different folks, but understand that you or you and your wife may know more than your physician or health care team about her condition and about what's working or not. There is a balance here that is important. A physician-patient relationship is a sacred trust where we literally put our lives in the hands of another person, but he/she is not God, despite our tendency to put them on a pedestal. They are human. They are pressured and hassled these days by the demands of managed care companies and regulators. They make mistakes. That is inevitable.

The key is to be aware, learn about your treatment to the point you can be a knowledgeable partner in decision making. I think often of my sister handling our father's treatment as a medical center in Maine. He was experiencing a very disagreeable and life threatening reaction to a medication. He was at his summer home, so this was a new cancer team, who were less familiar with the man we loved, though they were top clinicians. It was my sister's persistence, her understanding of his treatment and her tracking of that treatment, that allowed her to step in, literally identify the cause of his virtual dementia, and get the treatment changed, thus giving him another three and a half months of life, including some wonderful family time together on the coast of Maine.

Or Shirley speaking up when her treatment on the first day of radiation therapy was much less than sterling. Being docile or a grin and bear it approach is not good for you, nor ultimately for the hospital or cancer center providing your treatments. While a "good patient" as defined by health care professionals may cite compliance and other forms of infantilization, a good patient in our mind is one who with her family is actively involved in treatment and insisting on what is best for her and her family.

Mastectomy, Lumpectomy & Reconstruction

Mastectomy or lumpectomy? Choosing whether or not to have breast reconstruction or to use artificial breast prostheses? These are her very personal choices for her to make with the advice of her physician and perhaps some understanding of the experience of other women facing similar diagnoses and similar stages of cancer. You cannot make this for her, nor can the physician or physicians.

Our best advice, listen carefully to the pros and cons of either choice. Understand the nature of your disease, the likelihood of "getting it all" or not, or how important cleavage or decolletage is to her sense of self and her sense of femininity.

For myself, I remembered a former NBC reporter who had had a mastectomy without reconstruction describing herself as a 38-year-old woman on one side and an 8-year-old girl on the other. The description resonated with me, made it bearable or understandable, to the extent any man can truly understand.
Shirley is one of the one in twenty women choosing not to have reconstruction after her mastectomy, either at the time of the original surgery, or in subsequent years. Although unspoken, I believe deep in her soul she understood that her tumor and therefore cancer cells were still present in her chest. It was

better not to "stir them up" and live life fully with one breast and a prosthesis instead.

There are plenty of sources of lingerie and swim suits designed with mastectomy patients in mind, sometimes in specialized shops, and at other times in large department stores with a commitment to women who have had breast cancer surgery and treatment.

Sex After Breast Cancer

I have spoken on this subject to women's groups
and social workers. Most rewarding was being
part of a panel in Stamford, Connecticut with a
professional sex therapist speaking ahead of me.
I listened attentively and was pleased to find
that Shirley and I had figured out on our own
what she described in theory. She was a
theoretician explaining the principles underlying
sexuality and the impact of breast surgery and
cancer treatment. Shirley and I had lived it and
muddled through on our own just fine, thank
you.

This is another place where a man needs to let
his partner lead. She will let you know what
works now and what doesn't, what she's ready
for, and what she's not. I suppose I mourned
the loss of her breast as she did, as well as the
change in some aspects of love-making that
result.

The important thing to learn is that life goes on
and sex goes on. In the first weeks, months and
even years, your sex life may take on an added
dimension that is simultaneously painful and
exquisite. Imagine how it feels to make love to
someone you feel you might lose. You don't
want to hurt her. Remember, she is not fragile.
You can giver her bear hugs both during and
outside your lovemaking.

One of the best things for us was a marvelous gynecologist that discussed sexual issues with Shirley and had a number of practical suggestions. Most important was "the stuff used by prostitutes in Stamford" to be used by us to make intercourse more comfortable for her. A blessing. Yes there is both life and sex during and after treatment for breast cancer.

Alive

When you wake up in the morning, you know that it is a good day. When you turn one year older, including "big ones" like 40 and 50, you know you are having a good day. To this day, there are acquaintances who ask "How's Shirley" and I know they are prepared and almost expect to hear the worst. They mean well, but they are a reminder of what we faced together and what we had to overcome. Surprise, surprise, she is alive and well. Thank you!

Support Groups

I have been a strong advocate of support groups personally and professionally for more than 26 years. No matter what the situation or what the illness you are facing, it is profoundly comforting and helpful to be with others in comparable situations. You learn intellectually and spiritually that you are not alone.

In Shirley's case, two organization services were particularly beneficial and helpful: one, the Reach to Recovery program of the American Cancer Society, and, second, the Encore program of the YWCA. Reach to Recovery is a woman-to-woman visit by a former breast cancer patient to a woman facing or just having breast cancer surgery. In addition to helping with information and education, the mere site of a healthy survivor carries a strong message of hope.

While Reach to Recovery is short term, immediate support, YWCA Encore programs offer ongoing support groups that incorporate exercise, sometimes in a pool, sharing and discussing issues, and socialization. The two are a powerful combination. Another resource growing across the country is the Y-ME breast cancer organization, along with a myriad of national and local organizations fighting the disease, often with some form of education and support as part of their message and service.

Growth
Alison Flierl

She smiles at her little girl as she twirls through
the green grass
The tiny, pudgy legs intertwine and down she
goes on her bum
As the chubby cheeks mold into a pout, she
reaches out her arms
And scoops the giggling girl up into the sunny
air
A twinge of pain flies from under her arm to her
chest
And her memory reflects on aerobics and hard
mattresses

A deviation occurred in the message-like matter
This lone straggler separates from the group
And starts to grow unlike his many normal
companions
It makes new friends like itself, different from the
rest
They grow and grow

The summer passes, days of floating lazily on
the lake,
Days of lemonade and sun in the little one's hair
It is a normal time, despite the strained muscles
She must have accomplished during aerobics
Finally the time comes to go home and back to
reality.

These aberrances form their own society
Blacklisted from the normal way of life
They continue their growth and form quite a
group.
Each tick of the clock contributes to their strength
They grow and grow

The little one goes to her nursery school
Where she learns to build great ABC clock
structures
And that thou who has the most My Little Ponies
wins;
She goes back to teaching across the hall and
waits
There is uncertainty in the back of her mind, but
for now she waits.

The dark ones have now gained in number and
lunacy
They become plunderers of their weaker
neighbors
Taking and depriving them of what they need to
survive
Greed is their God and multitude their weapon...
They grow and grow

The face brightens under the white bangs; blue
eyes stare up
In wonder at the woman she loves and treasures
She runs downstairs leaving the woman to
contemplate
The pain that has not ceased and the worry that
has not abated
Finally, one day her mind suggests the terrible
possibility.

They continue their stealing and brute force
The innocent are killed or left in no state to live
And they are close to the shores
That will lead them to triumph and conquest,
They grow and grow.

Her shaking fingers search and find what they
fear most
An indignant, alien bit of hard tissue deep
within her breast.
She finds the strength to walk down to watch
the tiny one,
Her heart quakes with the thought of not being
able to continue
So finally she reaches for the phone.

The dark ones have found the shores they have
searched for
Yet they are not ready for the trip
They continue their actions of violence
And work on increasing their mass
They grow and grow.

The little one is dropped off for another day of
sandboxes and story books
While she is brought to the white, sterile
building
There they insert a needle to search and confirm
their suspicions
They find the intruders, and at once try to cut
them off from total victory
She is told of the weaponry they will continue to
use in this battle.

*They lose almost their whole army, yet there are
still a few
Who are strong and thirst for triumph, who make
it to the shores
There they set sail in hopes of ravaging all and
any who get in the way
They are weaker, but still have the strength of
insanity
They grow and grow*

Lines are drawn across her delicate skin and
then she is wheeled in
The laser, that's how she sees them, are pointed
at her body
During it all, she closes her eyes and dreams of
the little one
In the summer, rocking her at night, and of
hopes for future
And then they go on to fill her with illness

The dark ones are frightened but strong-willed
Many have died as of lately
But they continue to struggle upstream
Where they may be able to find success
They struggle to grow and grow.

Months pass, treatment continues, and she
sleeps for many hours
The little one makes creations with her crayolas
of love.
It is intense, and she grows more tired by the
day.
Yet her prayers intensify as does her love of life
Finally, they are done and it is time to wait.

They are dying, they know the smell of death
Usually it arises because of their exertions
Now those who once fed them have turned
against them
There is no hope unless one survives
They die and die.

More time passes and the little one grows a bit
less little.
Waiting provides comfort and safety in its lack of
events
She goes back to watching the white-haired girl
grow
And smiling at the giggles and shouts of
enthusiasm
As she twirls in the grass that is green once
again.

Scared
Alison Flierl

Here my baby lies secure in her dreams
While my head is filled with silent screams
I'm lying next to her, watching the small form
While it does my body unspeakable harm
My tears flow freely yet without noise
For in front of her I must hold my poise
She must never know the fear inside of me
Terror, that makes me tremble, she can never
see
Some people fear bugs, the dark
Or walking alone in an empty park,
Now I know what true fear is about
Being unable to see your child smile or pout
I might not be there for prom or another
special day
And all that could be left of me is a stone of gray
I can't leave yet, I'm going to fight
I will use every ounce of strength and might
I want to see my daughter grown
To see when boys start to call on the phone
I fear not being there for everything
For the prom dress and the wedding ring
I want to see it all, the good and bad
For her to have parents, not just Dad
How scared I am, as upon my child I gaze
Whom for I so wish to be there to help raise.

A Daughter's Letter Home

Hello Parents,

I'm writing to say thank you. I always know that I have fun parents who I love very much, but sometimes I take for granted how many opportunities you've given me. You've given me self esteem by always making me know I was your first priority. You've taught me love and strength and showed me what a good marriage is. You've allowed me to learn from your mistakes.

Dad, whenever you talk about drinking, you kind of roll your eyes and just talk about how stupid it was, but I find it amazing that you have been sober for this long and am so proud of the strength you have, and the wisdom you had to overcome something that just eats away at so many people's lives (especially here in L.A.).

Mom, you are one of my heroes. I don't always tell you how proud I am of your strength and bravery, but I should tell you more often. I am proud of you overcoming cancer and having an amazing attitude about it. I am proud of your "battle scar" and the inner strength it signifies.

You guys have given me a good outlook on life and all the bumps it will bring. You gave me a great school system, even though it cost a fortune to live in Greenwich. You let me go to a private college and even supported me when I chose to be a film major (other parents might say that is not practical). You've supported me when I've had these unpaid internships and never really complained about the extra stuff, let alone bills from college.

And though I probably won't be getting a red BMW convertible for my birthday (remember, I was promised whatever car I wanted for my 21st birthday—there is still time to pick one out...hee hee, just kidding). Seriously, though, I am so lucky at the opportunities you've made available to me and am lucky to have such supportive parents.

I hope to make you proud. I love you and miss you.

Your favorite daughter

**Are you looking for an inspirational or
motivational speaker for your next
conference or meeting?**

**Make your gathering exciting,
educational and meaningful!**

**Peter J. Flierl, MSW
brings your group experience
and expertise, including:**

Over 30 years in community health and wellness
A pioneer in complementary and alternative medicine

Topics such as:

*Prayer, Laughter & Broccoli
Sexuality & Breast Cancer
See the Miracle in the Mirror
Living Well to 125: Mind, Body & Spirit
Starting Over at 56
The Ten Percent Solution*

Peter Flierl would welcome the opportunity to
speak at your meeting or conference.

For information, call
(203) 273-5168 or 877-733-0528
or write to:
Witty Fools Productions
P.O. Box 481058
Los Angeles, California 90048

Give the Gift of Love.
Share experience, strength and hope.

Order extra copies of
Prayer, Laughter & Broccoli
Being There When Your Wife Has Breast Cancer

_Yes, I want ____ copies of *Prayer, Laughter & Broccoli* at $12.00 each
plus $1.25 Shipping & Handling per book. Allow 15 days for delivery.
_My check or money order for $_____ is enclosed.

Name_____

Address_____

_____

E-Mail _____

Mail TO – NAME _____

Address _____

_____
Please donate 10% of the purchase price to
_____

_____
Please make your check payable to Witty Fools
and return to:
Witty Fools Productions
P.O. Box 481058
Los Angeles, CA 90048

Or order by:
Toll-Free Phone 877-733-0528
Fax 203-637-1119
E-Mail: wittyfools@aol.com or fbtworld@aol.com
Thank you for your order.

We are compiling insights and tips for the next edition of **Prayer, Laughter & Broccoli** from other men in the lives of women living with breast cancer, and from women with a husband or partner who made a positive difference. We'd love to hear from you.....

Send your insights and tips to
Witty Fools
P.O. Box 481058
Los Angeles, California 90048-2633
wittyfools@aol.com